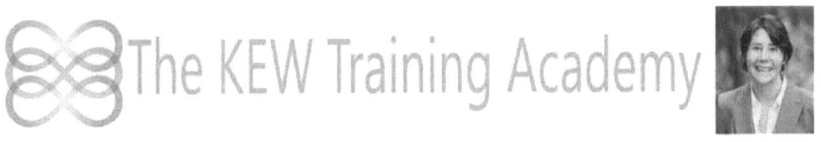

HYPNOSIS FOR CHILDBIRTH

ADVANCED HYPNOTHERAPY TECHNIQUES

THE KEW TRAINING ACADEMY LTD

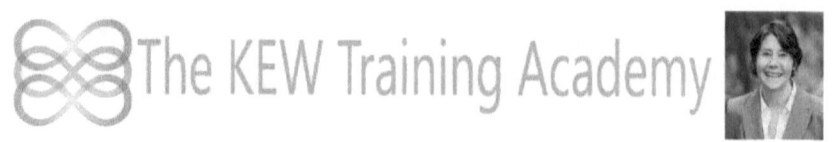

The KEW Training Academy Ltd

The KEW Training Academy was founded by Karen E Wells in 2006 and now offers many online & classroom courses enabling anyone to learn easy and effectively.

Karen has taught, and worked, widely in the UK, Europe, North America and Australia.

Email: hello@kewtraining.com

Website: www.kewtraining.com

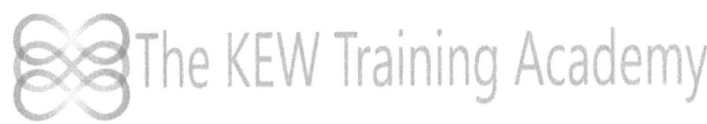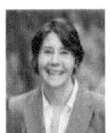

Welcome to Hypnosis for Childbirth

Online Learning Course

Welcome to your Hypnosis for Childbirth Online Learning Course.

This course is suitable for those that are already qualified in Hypnotherapy and wish to offer Hypnosis for Childbirth to their clients. It is also suitable for those that are pregnant and wish to undertake the journey of Self Hypnosis to help their birthing process. If you have purchased this course because you want to listen to the self hypnosis tracks to help you on your birthing process, please proceed to the video modules within the course itself. This training manual is for those that are experienced Hypnotherapists.

Your package contains the following:

The Training Modules – Two Modules taking you through each session with your client, as well as covering your consultation with them.

The Training Manual - An in depth look at Hypnosis for Childbirth. How this can help your client achieve the birth that they want and how you can help them. Also included are several scripts, along with a detailed account of when to do the sessions with your client during their pregnancy. Also included, if you wish to obtain a Diploma, are case review outlines and details of how to obtain your qualification and certification.

When you finish the course and provide me the required case reviews, I warmly look forward to welcoming you to The KEW Training Academy.

Klvns

Karen E Wells

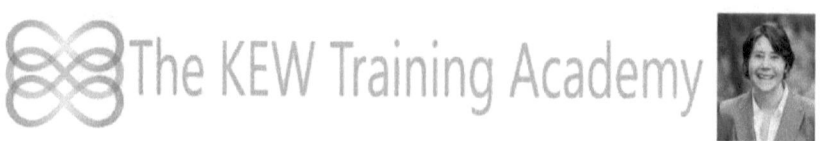

MODULE 1: THE CONSULTATION

Initial Contact With The Client

Your client may choose to contact you via a variety of methods, including telephone, email, text, to name but a few. It is always best to respond to your client promptly within your own working hours as you would do with a standard Hypnotherapy session. Much of your conversation will take place before the consultation, but there are a couple of fundamental things you need to find out from your client first of all. Have they experienced Hypnosis before? Why are they coming to you for this session and what is it that they would like to achieve from Hypnosis for Childbirth?

Contraindications/Suitability

Most clients that come to you are suitable for this programme. However, as with Hypnosis there are some contraindications to be aware of. People that are on anti–psychotic drugs, epileptic medication, schizophrenia medication or under the influence of alcohol or drugs etc are not suitable for this. The above is not an exhaustive list – please refer to the contraindications that are advised against with Hypnosis. Remember you are within your rights to refuse to do a session with a client if you do not feel it is the right time or the right thing to do. It is also within your rights to ask for a letter from their doctor to confirm they are suitable for these sessions.

The Right Time To Start Hypnosis For Childbirth Sessions

To start the Hypnosis for Childbirth sessions, ideally the client would be about 32 weeks in gestation. If the client wishes to start before then, avoid the first trimester.

The Appointment

When your client arrives for their appointment, there is likely to be a level of nervousness or anxiety about the upcoming sessions. This is the time to put them at ease. Better results come from sessions where you have a rapport with your client. Remember that they need to feel safe in your hands.

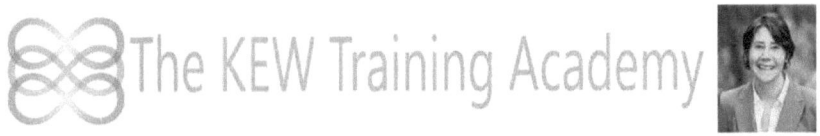

The Consultation/Pre-Talk

This is one of the most important aspects of the whole session. It is during this time that you will find out all about your client, why they are here, what they want to achieve, have they experienced Hypnosis before? Here is one part where you do a lot of talking! It is very important to explain to your client about Hypnosis – what it is, what it isn't and to manage their expectations.

In the Consultation you will discuss the following:

Managing Expectations

It is so important to manage your client's expectations on so many levels. Your client may have concerns about whether this will truly help them and to what degree. After all, childbirth can be daunting whether the client has experienced it before or not. Let your client know they are in safe hands.

Time Limits

How long will your sessions for Hypnosis for Childbirth be?

Typically, as with standard Hypnosis, the first session will be the longest. This is where you will gain all the information from your client so you should allow 1½ hours for the first session and 1 hour for subsequent sessions should be adequate.

Example of Consultation/Pre-Talk Form

The following page shows an example of the Consultation/Pre-talk form. Feel free to add to it or amend any information to suit you.

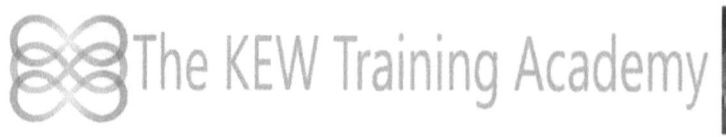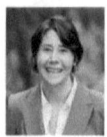

CONSULTATION FORM

Full Name ....

Date ....

Address ....

Age ....

Marriage Status ....

Any other Children? ....

Occupation ....

Tel no ....

Email Address ....

Are you currently taking any medication? ....

Have you ever had psychiatric treatment? ....

Have you any physical/medical condition other than your pregnancy?

....

If so, are you consulting your GP on this matter? ....

What are your reasons for wanting to experience Hypnosis for Childbirth?

....

....

....

What would be your ideal birth plan? (How, where, medication)

....

.

How many weeks of Gestation are you presently?

....

Any other information you wish to let me know?

....

Your Signature ....

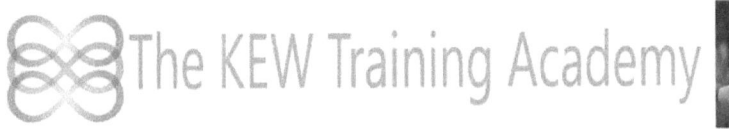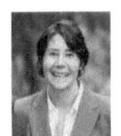

MODULE 1 ACTION POINTS:

☐ Design your own Hypnosis for Childbirth consultation form. What, if anything would you change?

Once completed, you are ready to move on to Module 2: The Hypnosis for Childbirth Sessions.

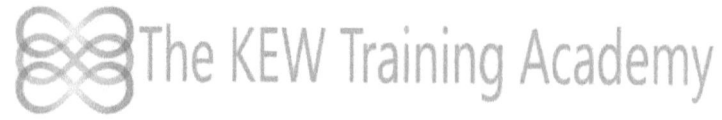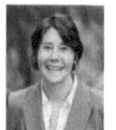

MODULE 2: THE HYPNOSIS FOR CHLDBIRTH SESSIONS

The Order Of The Sessions

With the Hypnosis for Childbirth programme, you should schedule three sessions with the client for maximum results.

They will be as follows:

Session 1)

General Relaxation Session: This is a session that you will create for your client so they get used to your voice and the levels of relaxation needed for the sessions. Put some suggestions in this session along the lines of: "And each time you hear my voice, you will relax even more deeply, the connection with your body will increase and you will trust yourself to have the birth experience that you want".

Session 2)

Pain Management Sessions: At the end of this module, you will find the scripts for three Pain Management sessions. Choose one of these to practice with your client in this session. Record a CD/MP3's with these three sessions on and give to the client to practice from now until the day they give birth.

Session 3)

Pre-Childbirth Session: This will be the session that you do with the client which you will record and send to the client as a CD/MP3. They will listen to this once a day from this session until the day before labour begins. They can alternate it with the Pain Management sessions if necessary.

You will then give a recording to your client of a MP3/CD that they will listen to once labour has started (This is the Childbirth Day Recording). This can be on repeat for as long as the labour/birth lasts.

It is best to schedule the live sessions one or two weeks apart from each other.

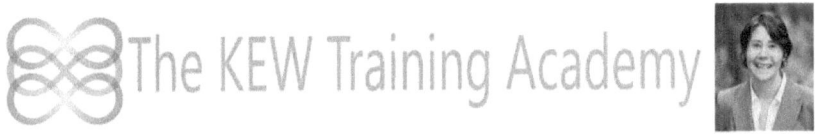

Session 1: Relaxation Session

As stated, this is the first session that you will do with your client. Create a relaxation session for them of approximately 25 minutes long that will include the suggestions: "And each time you hear my voice, you will relax even more deeply, the connection with your body will increase and you will trust yourself to have the birth experience that you want".

Give the recording of this session to your client so they get used to your voice and to the levels of relaxation needed for the sessions and their birth experience.

Session 2: Pain Management Sessions

There are three Pain Management sessions that you will give your client as recordings for them to listen to in their own time. For best results, the client will listen to one or all of these recordings once a day from the day of the session with you until the birth of their child.

The scripts are at the end of this module but here is a description of each Pain Management session.

General Pain Control Induction: This gives the client the suggestion that their pain is like a tunnel that they can enter and exit, seeing the light ahead.

Anaesthesia Switch: The suggestion here is that there is a switch behind the client's neck that goes down the spinal column. They visualise a dimmer switch which controls the amount of anaesthesia that goes into the body.

Glove Anaesthesia: The client is given the suggestion that one of their hands is in a bucket of ice cold water that numbs the hand and they are able to place it to any part of their body that feels sore or needs some pain relief.

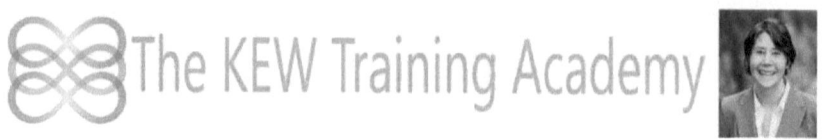

Session 3: Pre-Childbirth Session

This is the session that will lead your client up to the day before labour begins. It's a beautiful session connecting the client with the unborn baby and visualising it coming into the world.

You will give your client this as a recording so they can listen to it every day leading up to the birth. They can also alternate it with listening to the Pain Management sessions.

Session 4: Childbirth Day

This session will not be done with the client as a live session for obvious reasons but will be given as a recording on the final session that you do with the client. As you give them the recording, make the client aware that they can play this as soon as labour starts and they can play it on repeat for as long as the labour and birth last. It is also a good idea for your client to let their midwife know that they will be quite relaxed as they will be in Hypnosis for the duration of the labour and birth.

You may wish to create a Hypnosis for Childbirth package for your client, offering them three live Hypnotherapy sessions and a series of recordings.

You are also able to offer sessions to groups for Hypnosis for Childbirth.

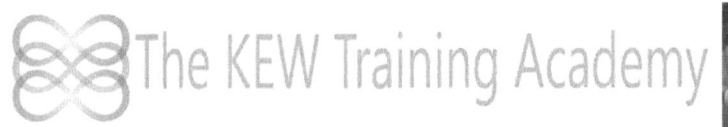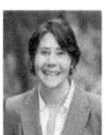

MODULE 3: PAIN MANAGEMENT SCRIPTS

These are the scripts for use with your client for the Pain Management Sessions. Please note that you must include an Induction & Deepener of approx. five to ten minutes before bringing in the following scripts and suggestions.

General Pain Control:
Now I want you to take the pain and give it a shape and a form. As you do this, make it into a tunnel, a tunnel that you can easily enter and exit at your own will.....now imagine, sense or feel yourself entering that tunnel and as you enter it, the intensity of your pain increases for just a moment.....and that is ok.....you can see a light at the end of this tunnel and as you walk through the tunnel, every step you take takes you away from the pain and discomfort and so the deeper into the tunnel you go, the less pain and discomfort you feel.....the light at the end of the tunnel grows larger and larger and as it grows larger and larger, you begin to feel better and better......each step reducing your pain and discomfort..... each step healing and strengthening your body.......with every step you feel more comfortable......so much more comfortable......and as you reach that light at the end you feel relieved of any pain or any discomfort.....feeling relaxed, strong and comfortable.... and so from now on, each time you enter this tunnel and pass through the tunnel, you watch the light at the end get stronger, and you get stronger.....this tunnel is yours, you control it and as you exit the tunnel you feel better and better, stronger and stronger and passing through it will always make you feel better.

Anaesthesia Switch:
Guiding your client back into Hypnosis, continue as follows:

I would like you to imagine that a switch is placed behind your neck and that switch goes down all the way down the spinal column. This switch, when it's off, creates a large amount of numbness from just below your breasts to just above your knees. You also now visualise a dimmer switch that you can adjust to create the level of Anaesthesia that you require....You know that you have complete control to adjust the level and to adjust the dimmer switch so by focusing on adjusting the dimmer switch to any area of your body you have complete control to adjust the level and the intensity of comfort that you want.....

You have complete control for specific comfort and sensation levels. You're able to control and regulate, whereby you feel pressure but not discomfort and this allows you to be able to time your contractions so at the onset of labour you will do.......All the nerves from just above your knees.... front and back, your pubic area, buttocks, abdomen, lower and upper back and chest to just below your breasts......If you now visualise this area like a barrel from just below your breasts to just above your knees and circling your body......By adjusting the dimmer dial to the appropriate level of Anaesthesia and comfort..... you can make this where you feel pressure and movement but no discomfort...... pressure and movement but no discomfort and whenever you switch it off, then it's off.... believe it.....accept it and at any point you need to move then you can turn off this switch off and when you're settled again switch it to the on position......you have total control.......

Glove Anaesthesia:
Guiding your client back into Hypnosis:

And as you continue to relax I want you to imagine that one of your hands is in a bucket of ice cold water.......so cold that you can practically feel the imaginary ice cubes bumping into your hand.........and at first you notice a little discomfort and then gradually a numb tingling sensation in the fingertips........ which creeps up into your whole hand and you imagine your hand in that bucket of cold chilling ice water.........the colder, the number your hand will become....... and you really notice that coldness, that numbness develop.......... this numbness in your hand becoming numb and wooden like....... Becoming more number and wooden-like............... when it feels so cold and numb you slowly and gently allow your hand to lift towards the left side of your face..............as your hand slowly but surely moves towards the left side of your face it becomes much more wooden and numb.....noticing that the closer it approaches your left cheek the number it becomes....... and when it finally reaches your left cheek you let the palm of your hand rest lightly against your cheek........ and allow the numbness to be transferred from your palm to the left side of your cheek........

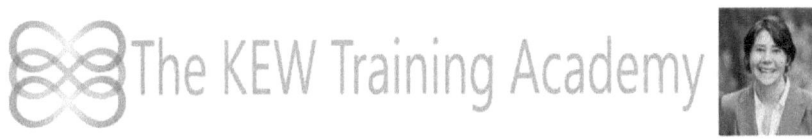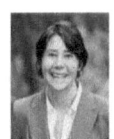

When you're certain that your cheek has become so very numb....... being certain of the coldness and numbness onto the left side of your face.............. only then will your hand drop to your side and your hand will return to feel normal........... however the left side of your face will feel just as if the dentist has injected something into your gums..... and as you remember that feeling in your gums how leathery and stiff it is now on one side of your face....how it feels following an injection....... so now whenever you're ready you can gradually bring yourself out of hypnosis and as you do this numbness remains on the left side of your face for two minutes and then returns to normal..... so you can open your eyes and feel the numbness there now on the left side of your face.......

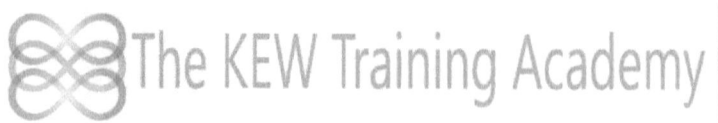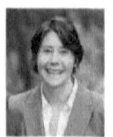

MODULE 4: PRE-CHILDBIRTH DAY SCRIPT

I want you to understand consciously and subconsciously that each and every time you play this recording it will be fantastic practice for your childbirth. And when you listen you are resting comfortably now.......paying close attention to my voice and imagining yourself on the day when you're going to give birth to your child...... you'll be able to make all the necessary phone calls and arrangements that have been agreed upon to obtain assistance in your baby's delivery....... I'm going to help you to become so deeply relaxed that you can accept any suggestions to make that birthing easier so you can choose to listen or not listen and you can stop this process any time you want by simply counting up from 1 to 5.......

You're the one that is in control at all times but first I'm going to ask you to relax in two ways physically and then mentally and both are as important as each other because when your mind and body are really relaxed you have a door opened to the subconscious part of your mind..... where you have all the benefits of yourself......now make sure now that you're in a comfortable position and that you're taking a long deep breath, breathing out slowly..... allowing your eyes to close, relaxing all the muscles and when you're so sure that they're so relaxed that they won't open even if you tried and you can test them now to notice how good that feels that you let that relaxation go from your eyes all the way down to the tips of toes......

Feel the relaxation flowing through your body..... letting go and you allow the sound of my voice to guide you deeper and deeper, relaxed.... so the more relaxed you are, the better you feel and the better you feel, the more relaxed you become..... so now let's see if you can allow this physical part of you to relax even more..... so in a moment I will ask you to slowly open and then close your eyes..... when you close your eyes you send a deep wave of relaxation through your body so that instantly the physical part of you grows twice as deeply relaxed and you can make that happen very quickly...... now slowly let your eyes open and close your eyes and now feel a powerful wave of relaxation moving down through your body..... letting go of everything now....... feeling your body relax......

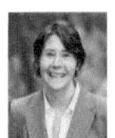
In this warm safe blanket of relaxation...... from this moment on every gentle breath you exhale helps you to relax even deeper....... so moving back to your mind to relax just as beautifully as your body is relaxed...... and when your mind is relaxed that's when you have your mind open to the subconscious....... when you can take on board all the help for the loving joyous birth without any discomfort...... so here's how you can have that mental relaxation..... in a moment I'm going to ask you to slowly begin counting backwards from 100 but I want you to see the numbers in your mind's eye before you say it so I want you to visualise the number 100 say to yourself 100 and then say deeper relaxed so with each number you say.......deeper relaxed.......

Can you now let your mind go twice as relaxed with a wonderful, calm feeling.... you are drifting deeper as you say this to yourself..... then you see the next number 99 before you say it..... and again deeper relaxed...... and an interesting thing happens..... each number become smaller and fainter than the one before..... so it follows in a very short time that the numbers are so small and so faint you just can't find them........ this happens very quickly....... relaxing all of the numbers out of your mind ....at about 87 when you can't find that number....... you are so marvellously relaxed..... so if you already see that number 100 saying deeper relaxed...... 99 deeper relaxed...... and relax those numbers right out of your mind....... now begin to let the numbers go smaller and more distant letting them drift further away........

Let them drift away now relaxing..... then when they are all gone...... so you feel so good now ....your mind relaxed...... your body is relaxed...... and your mind and your body can relax much more with every gentle breath you exhale....... I want you to know that each and every time you enter a state of relaxation you will go in easier, faster, deeper......

Each and every time you enter a state of relaxation you enter it easier, faster, deeper..... that's the way the mind works..... deeper and deeper into relaxation ......seeing yourself calm relaxed confident and strong....... just resting there and imagining your mind....watching a video presentation of the progress of your pregnancy and the time ahead projecting your thoughts forward in time....... and seeing the birth experience with the correct future time and date ....

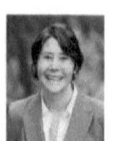
Starting from now........ seeing yourself walking and talking playing a joyful and active part in the ongoing living reality...... taking time out now to rest, relax, happily, energetic and strong confident and self-assured.......... deeply enjoying every moment of now....... your experience of childbearing bringing a joyous intensity into your daily life....... A purpose in this miraculous experience of life....... this life we are all here to celebrate...... you and your child choosing to share....... and now as you relax more deeply with each gentle breath that you take see yourself making all the arrangements, clarifying all the plans with everyone privileged to be involved..... seeing yourself on the video screen of the time and the date chosen by nature as the first stage of labour begins and it seems that you have shown you have known sometime ahead that this would be the day........

And you see yourself smiling, breathing easily...... fully in control....... as the plans unfold......... for your body really knows what to do....... there is no need to remind yourself to breathe........ no need to remind your heart to beat....... your body really does know what to do....... you relax...... you have prepared yourself well for this moment....... free from stress, strain or discomfort........ you have no cares or worries right now ....all your cares and worries just drift away...........

Imagine a fluffy cloud above you, floating across the sky....... you allow yourself to put in any of your nervous feelings on the cloud and allow it to drift away into the distance...... further and further away....... so far and so distant that you really notice it now......allowing it to be just a dot on the horizon......And you do not let it totally disappear because you because you may choose to retain these feelings and retrieve them if you need them.......... right now you have no need for them......... you let them go and as you do, you gain a sense of peace and calm flowing within your body....... you are peaceful, calm and relaxed...... you go deeper and deeper......deeper and deeper....... and as I talk to you, you continue to go into even deeper state of relaxation......... my voice is becoming remote now....... nothing else but my voice is important....... nothing else is important...... nothing else but my voice....... when I say to you...... right now seems of interest...... even though my voice may come to you from a distance or it may change in quality....... my voice travels along with you and it doesn't matter where you go........ my voice will go along with you as you relax more and more........ relaxing deeper and deeper into this wonderful relaxed state...... you're bearing a child , feeling the movement within you .....

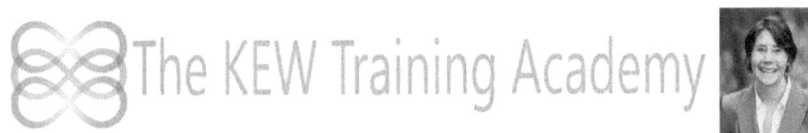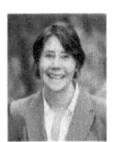

Growing..... preparing for entry into this world..... you give birth to your baby with joy and relaxation....... this process is a natural and automatic one, in which you will be relaxed and you know that you are courageous and strong...... saying this will be a reminder to yourself to enhance your ongoing health and healing process of your body......... and you can see yourself on the day when you're going to give birth to your child...... calm, relaxed, confident........ feeling really strong and courageous....... you'll be able to adjust yourself to your environment...... even though you cannot change it...... you can do everything better when you're relaxed...... whether it be physical, mental or emotional...... instantly you're going to be aware that with each contraction you will feel the pressure of the contraction but the feeling is never going to become discomfort...... it's always going to be a feeling of comfort of complete relaxation.......

You can control your entire body with your mind..... you are relaxed and you have the ability to deliver your child in peace and relaxation....... you know the birth of your child is going to be a joyful event in your life....... you will be alert to hear your baby's first cry...... there is joy in you and you feel strong and courageous and there's an inner strength in your entire being...... a feeling of strength and confidence and vitality...... you allow yourself to sink into an even deeper state of relaxation as you'll be able to control and maintain harmony within your body..... you will be able to easily effortlessly and naturally....numb yourself in various areas just by imagining walking into a cold lake, your body becomes so cold and numb....... all the way to the top of your breasts....... so cold and numb and even picturing the on and off switch and the dimmer switch being able to turn the switch off easily......

And use the dimmer switch to turn down any discomfort......this gives you complete control to adjust your body...... your comfort level and anaesthaesia level...... you have complete control to adjust the level and to turn the switch to off ....to produce numbness so you find the area above your breasts, to just above your knees and circling your body you have complete control now to obtain the level of comfort that you want........ you have complete control and you can regulate the degree of dullness whereby you feel pressure but no discomfort.......

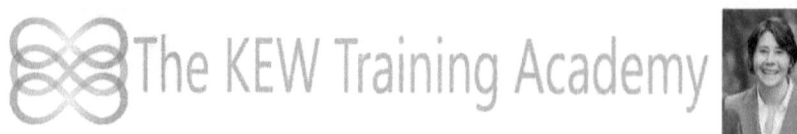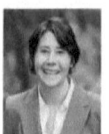

You're going to have contractions but they are going to be something nice to happen...... you will feel pressure only in a pleasant way as each contraction takes you nearer and nearer to the birth of your baby.......

Wherever your partner's hand is that touches any part of your body and says the word RELAX......you will drift 10 times deeper..... so easily...... so automatically.....and produce more anaesthetic, creating the required amount.......the desired amount of numbness...... feeling pressure and movement but no discomfort........

You notice your contractions will be increasingly becoming more frequent and you'll be able to adjust the level of dumbness by adjusting the dimmer switch to the reduced level of intensity of sensation to various parts of your body.......achieving the amount of sensation needed to feel the pressure and movement on a comfortable level...... so you can help your baby come out when you are dilated to 1 cm you notice the air becoming cooler and by 10 cm you feel wonderfully cool and calm........

Confident and strong minded you allow yourself to go into an even deeper state of relaxation so that you may help yourself and your baby to arrive safely...... becoming happier as you are getting closer and closer to your goal of delivering the baby....... and this will encourage you to gain all your strength....... to go deeper and deeper into hypnosis to help yourself and your baby........ being able to push your baby into the world...... allowing yourself to go into a very relaxed state....... deeper than you ever experienced before...... by allowing yourself to go into this state, you permit your body to flow in its natural rhythm to help and assist the natural movement of your muscles......... like the natural gentle rhythm of movement as you allow yourself to go deeper and deeper and become more and more relaxed.......

You are so relaxed that at the point you need to, you are able to push your baby out into the world....... with peace and tranquility........ time passes quickly and pleasantly........ and there is no fatigue, nausea or exhaustion....... because of your relaxation, your birthing advances with each contraction.....You are allowing yourself to sink deeper and deeper as each contraction means you're reaching your goal...... coming closer and closer to the welcoming of your child........ being able to move around....... you find a comfortable position, using the toilet if needed but still remaining deeply hypnotised.......

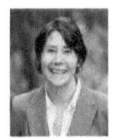

n fact you go deeper and deeper during the process of birthing than ever before.......
pening your eyes will not bring you back to your usual state of awareness but rather it will
llow you to sink even deeper and deeper into this wonderful state of relaxation...............

want you to practice this now remaining wonderfully beautifully deeply relaxed .... very,
ery slowly open your eyes...... just a little bit...... noticing how deeply relaxed you remain as
ou slowly open your eyes...... a bit more relaxed...... when you're ready you can close your
yes and relax 10 times deeper........ feeling really good, aware of any sounds and noises
round you...... any sounds will not disturb you instead they act as the signal to deepen your
ypnosis.......easily able to relax.......

o that you know yourself you can feel pressure and movement but no discomfort...... your
ody gently easing your child into the ideal birth position........ enjoying every new moment of
his profound exhilarating and emotional experience....... resting in the intervals between
ontractions........ plenty of time for preparations or arrangements ....all part of your well
ade plans...... being responsive..... calm..... centred...... fully in control........ focusing on
our breathing....... feeling vibrant, strong, feeling really good and wonderful........ you and
our child responding as one to the signals of life....... reassuring your child....... sharing
hese feelings....... your loving thoughts and emotions and relaxing........ appreciating the
enefit of these weeks of preparation and expert advice all those around you now playing
heir part with sensitivity.......

s your contractions become more frequent, you're able to relax easier than you ever
hought possible...... trusting your body...... being in control...... aware of the support around
ou...... flowing in the rhythm of life....... as you drift down relaxing...... feeling flexible,
omfortable, calm ....you know that your child knows exactly when to be born......

ou know your child knows exactly how to be born.......... a tiny head leading the way easing
own your birth canal coming gently into life........ to love ....to your arms........ beautiful,
ealthy, happy newborn child...... feeling the strength of the ability within yourself......
njoying the unique splendour of your being...... just being you........

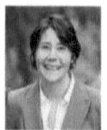
This wonderful process of bringing life and love to the world...... your daily ability to relax deeply is preparing you well for the birth of your child....... preparing you for saving your energy to welcome your child........ a wonderful happy event and during the birth experience you find time to appreciate and respond to the expert and sensitive help and advice that you receive........ finding it easy to tune out any comments and sounds that might otherwise distract you from focusing fully on this creative purpose.........

Your energy, endurance and strength will be more than equal to the need....... your mind and body able to cope effortlessly with any eventuality......

And you know the opening your eyes will not bring you back to your usual state of awareness....... it allows you to relax even deeper....... and when the delivery team announce that your baby is being born.......... you will be able to open your eyes to touch and assist your baby coming out into this world....... watching the birth of the baby with interest ....you can really notice all of your baby's features......... the eyes, nose, mouth and body, feeling a strong bonding taking place immediately...... easily picturing everything going smoothly and well....... feeling relaxed and if you need to in any area you can numb that with the exercises that you've practised...... and after giving birth you will feel only pleasantly tired....... so you can relax, sleeping easily at any time you feel the need..... feeling wonderful.

So whether you have a vaginal or Caesarean birth you're able to cope easily with all situations...... being flexible, saying to yourself...... I see myself birthing beautifully..... calmly and with confidence....... I deserve a fast, easy and completely comfortable birth.....my body knows how to give birth and I will let it....... my body will give birth in its own time....... birth is a completely easy and natural experience...... my body was designed for it........ giving birth in peace and calmness ....a joyful event......

You permit time for yourself to take naps when your body feels fatigued...... feeling a sense of power...... control..... inner strength....... taking control of your life...... feeling happy, healthy and seeing yourself more attractive than ever before......... and experiencing feeling the wonders of childbirth and every sensation before during and after feeling calm relaxed and in control.........

RING OUT OF HYPNOSIS

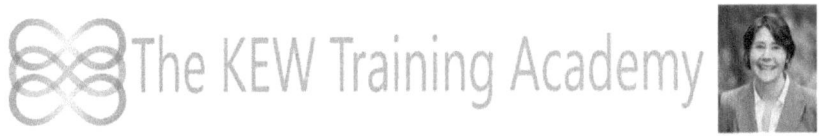

MODULE 5: CHILDBIRTH DAY SCRIPT

So settle yourself down now in any position that is comfortable for you....... just cooperate with the sound of my voice and settle yourself into a comfortable position and listen quietly to the sound of my voice....... taking in a deep breath....... and as you breathe out slowly...... closing your eyes and relaxing inside....... imagining any way that you can your eyes becoming very heavy and tired....... and you just quietly relaxing inside....... allow that relaxed feeling to go from your eyes all the way down to the tips of your toes....... the sound of my voice sends you deeper into relaxation & allows any sounds around you to deepen that relaxation........ as you enter this hypnotic state you simply allow yourself to go much deeper than at any time before...... know that you can turn your switch to the off position...... it is totally off........

The parts of your body from just above your knees........ front and back..... completely surrounding you........ every nerve, every muscle, so relaxed....... becoming deeply anaesthetised...flooding your body just as if you walk into a very cold Lake..... holding onto the jetty as you go slowly......... noticing the coldness ....coldness becoming numbness and the anaesthesia will become even more powerful with every breath you exhale to that part of your body...... so that when the time comes and your water breaks....... instantly when this happens a beautiful peace and serenity flows to your abdomen...... and your anaesthesia becomes powerfully stronger...... physical body letting go and dilating enough for your baby to come down and out into the world...... very quickly and easily to join you......and today you will be aware of things going on around you....... having a new belief system that you can and will control your mind and body..........The way nature intended from your first contraction......... feeling a wave of peace and tranquility and relaxation flowing through you.......

Because with each and every contraction this becomes so pleasant...... that with the third or fourth contraction you actually begin smiling and looking forward to the next one......

As you say that you are much nearer to the birth of your baby....... and with each contraction instantly you know you're in charge of this beautiful event........ no one is going to control it but you.........

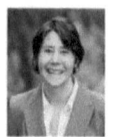

Instantly you're going to be aware that with each contraction your feel the pressure of the contractions but the feeling is never going to be discomfort....... it is always going to be a feeling of comfort...... of complete relaxation...... your body relaxes even more as it becomes more calm and peaceful...... relaxed...... you say to yourself you are prepared and ready for this beautiful birthing.......

The more contractions you have, the more anaesthesia is released into your body...... and if you want to........ need to........ you are able to walk and move into a more comfortable position but the middle part of you will remain completely and deeply anaesthetised ......so you now even relax even more and I am going to count from 10 all the way down to 0 and with each number you will have a powerful wave of relaxation through your mind and body so by the time I reached account of zero..........

Mentally and physically you have drifted 10 times deeper....... and your anaesthesia is much more powerful......... you want that.......you can have it....... very easily now...... 10 relaxation and anaesthesia deepening........ 9 wave of relaxation now......... 8 all the way down your body........7 letting go just drifting now throughout your mind and body...........

6 is even more powerful now as you drift downwards into your mind and body...... 5 mind and body becoming more calm & serene and peaceful....... 4 drifting down....... 3.....deeper and deeper mentally and physically......... 2 another powerful wave of relaxation........ 1 relaxation all the way down your body clearing your mind........... 0 that's good 10 times deeper into relaxation and anaesthesia .... just as if the middle part of your body had been totally and utterly relaxed and that relaxation penetrating every muscle, every fibre of your body now..........

You see the number 100 clearly in your mind and then you say to yourself..... deeper relaxed...... 99 deeper relaxed...... watch those numbers begin to fade...... going further away, going quickly now........ gone and as you listen you are aware of your surroundings.....you hear sounds around you that are perfectly normal...... and anything that sounds around you does not disturb you in any way...... the sounds help you to relax even more and take you deeper....... the only sounds that you allow yourself to be interested in is the sound of my voice guiding you deeper and deeper relaxed......

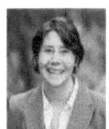
You put all of your nervous feelings about the baby's health….. fear of what people think…… doubts about yourself….. concern about your partner and any other negative thoughts to be placed on that cloud and allow it to drift far away into the distance……

Far away, further and further away…… so far and so distant that you barely notice it allowing it to be a dot on the horizon…… however you do not let it totally disappear because you may choose to retain these feelings and retrieve them if you need them…… right now you have no need for them…… you let them go and as you do you get a sense of peace and calm flowing within your body……. you can allow yourself the pleasure watching these feelings go further and further away and now you're peaceful calm and relaxed you go deeper and deeper as I talk to you…… and you continue to go into an even deeper state of relaxation……

Where everything but the sound of my voice is becoming remote now…… nothing else but my voice seems important and my voice will travel along with you…… and it doesn't matter where you go my voice goes with you……. my voice flows and travels along with you……. so that you will always continue to respond to me on a subconscious level……

So relax and while your powerful subconscious mind links in with the sound of my voice, you relax more and more….. you allow yourself to sink deeper and deeper into this wonderful state of peace and comfort……. where time passes quickly and pleasantly as you relax more and more……. you allow yourself to sink into a deep state of relaxation……. as one part of your body and your mind continues to focus on the heaviness of your arms and legs……..

You are in control of creating a comfortable environment so that you can turn your attention inwardly……. after all it's your inner experience of yourself that matters the most right now ……..to create a new opportunity taking in new ideas and finding ways to make use of them…….you are the one that is in control…… aware of your attention……. where it wanders too …….Physical mental or emotional……. I'd like to take another part of your mind to help you imagine that very special place…… an important place of yours to drift to it now and the nature of the conscious mind is such

23 | Page

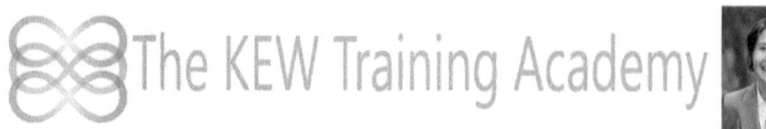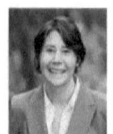

that it would naturally drift from here to your safe place......... and perhaps to nowhere in particular......... and whatever your conscious mind drifts to at any moment is just fine...... when you notice the routine sounds of the environment........ of your own thoughts of your own reactions to the different things that I say........

It could be very comforting to know that each contraction will make you feel more relaxed with a powerful wave of relaxation through your mind and body........ that is the nature of the mind drifting in and out....... and it can accept easily the different possibilities the part of you that is infinitely more interesting and powerful........ is your subconscious part of you that can listen and respond even when your conscious mind drifts elsewhere........ and your own subconscious mind has abilities that your conscious mind sometimes forgets about....... and when you're conscious of your subconscious mind's abilities to provide comfort during each and every contraction smiling and looking forward to the birth of your baby......

You are very relaxed and you can appreciate the comfort of recognising that with each contraction a wave of relaxation goes to your whole body from the top of your head down to the tips of your toes........ how the mind and the body can work so closely together sometimes when that's important and help other times the conscious mind and the subconscious mind can drift off elsewhere........ and the mind's greatest ability is the freedom to go where ever imagination wills it......

It's so much easier you can be so much more comfortable....... resting yourself so much more comfortably when your mind is there..... when your body is here....... it's just enough distance to be much more comfortable than you thought you could be and you can be very aware of that interesting sensation of being separate from your body of having all of yourself in the experience of deep hypnosis........... and you know and I know that as distant as your body feels on one level it feels close enough on another level to be aware of its need to continue to breathe in and slowly ....effortlessly........ comfortably....... as you're mind continues to float there and your body continues to rest comfortably over here.......... the conscious mind can certainly be curious about the comfortable sensations you are feeling........ the separation existing and you don't have to analyse to carefully know which part of you is the most comfortable at this moment...... you could simply allow yourself instead to enjoy the comfort that goes with the letting go of your mind........

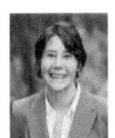
Not having to think and accept easily the different possibilities of what your conscious mind is capable of......... processing whatever it happens to notice........ the part of you that is infinitely more interesting and powerful is your subconscious part of you....... that can listen and respond even when your conscious mind is elsewhere....... your body instinctively knows what to do although you are deep within....... you are not alone......comforted by the presence of the support team....... this beautiful process of birthing transforms time......

Every 20 minutes seems like five minutes to you and your birthing goes by quickly and easily....... passing time proceeds very quickly and easily for you and even if you realise that a midwife or doctor needs to examine you..... check your dilation, or should you need to you can go to the toilet ....you can do this easily and remain wonderfully calm......

Remaining in that deep relaxed state the child you are bearing....... the child is developing...... growing and preparing for entry in this world and you're going to have to choose your to have your baby in absolute comfort with a wonderful feeling of joy....... you are able to give birth to baby with joy and relaxation much easier than you ever thought possible........ you have felt the movement of your child with the growing and developing.......

Preparing for entry into this world you give birth to a baby with joy relaxation...... the process is natural and automatic ....one in which you will be relaxed and know that you are strong and courageous....... you be able to adjust yourself to your environment even though you cannot change .... you can become more comfortable and you can do everything better when you are relaxed whether it be physical mental or emotional....... you're able to control your entire body within your mind ....you are relaxed and you deliver your child in peace and relaxation.........

As time passes quickly and pleasantly the act of childbirth will be as natural and as easy as any other process......... you allow your body to flow rhythmically...... feeling comfortable...... calm...... relaxed and courageous....... you know you're feeling strong and relaxed....... you know the birth of your child is a joyful event in your life....... feeling the calm.... relaxing sensations going throughout your entire body and that it is from your toes to the top of your head.......

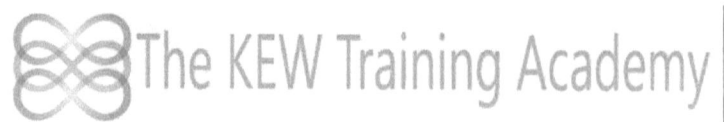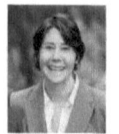

And you will be alert to hear your baby's first cry...... you are relaxed and peaceful...... courteous ......composed...... confident...... this joy and you feel strong and courageous and have an inner strength in your entire being......

At any point you may feel pressure and movement but no discomfort...... you notice your contractions are getting more frequent...... strong and efficient....... your uterus is very strong...... you actually begin smiling and looking forward to the next one....... as you say I am near to the birth of my baby........ and with each contraction your contractions feel like only pressure to you........ you are able to adjust the level of dullness by adjusting the dimmer switch to the level of intensity of sensation to the various parts of your body....... allowing you to discover that comfortable numbness

You now feel safe and secure.........as you relax, your cervix becomes softer and softer with each contraction....... that dilates you quickly and easily........ visualising your cervix opening up...... the more you're progressing to the end of your birthing confidence feeling every cell...... every muscle...... gaining in confidence....... birthing is a calm joyous event...... you and your body...... you and your baby working in complete harmony........ if it any time you need a supply of endorphins to increase your physical relaxation your mind supplies these they are already in your bloodstream........ your partner can massage you and when this happens very strong and powerful endorphins flow around your body relaxing you.......

The longer and stronger your contractions become the stronger and deeper your anaesthesia becomes....... feeling peaceful.......calm..... relaxed...... drifting..... floating...... you're doing so well...... calm...... comfortable...... relaxed while being monitored...... going to the bathroom.......relaxed.....

Having the baby's position checked and your dilation measured...... changing positions....... keeping the switch off and saying to yourself feeling pressure but no discomfort........ and if your attention is needed any time you are able to communicate....... and then drift back into a deeper relaxation........ this is accepted on all levels within you so that you help your baby...........

A number of things may develop and you can be flexible enough and appreciate them and fit them into the goal that you wish to achieve......... so if you need to hear what others are discussing you or your baby's progress in a way that is not beneficial.......

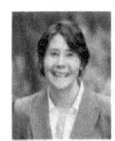

The KEW Training Academy

This will be a signal for you to go even deeper......... their voices will be muted...... white noise to your ears....... other noises around you will not disturb you....... instead they just calm and relax you........ and ask act as a signal to deepen your relaxation ....you remain calm relaxed confident and strong and you will if needed be able to instruct the delivery team through your ability to separate body from mind......... so that your body will feel totally heavy and then in a deep state of relaxation but able to respond in a very logical and appropriate manner to help you and your baby.......... and time passes quickly every 10 minutes seems like one minute........ you accomplish this....... so easily able to go on concentrating on a safe place.......

You forget to notice how much time goes by........ you relax even deeper........ time goes so quickly and you concentrate on the movement of your baby....... you commit yourself to take greater control by saying to yourself....... and your mind...... that you're calm relaxed confident and strong ....this permits you to drift into a very deep state of relaxation where you feel pressure and movement but no discomfort...... if there is need for any forceps or epidural, or to have a Caesarian because of the medical need for you or your baby......... this is a signal to reach an even deeper state and by doing so you are helping yourself and your baby......... remaining calm and acting appropriately........ help yourself and your baby and if there's any point in the process where you need to have an injection or infusion you can numb the area by focusing your mind....... noticing that you dilate beautifully and quickly........ naturally to the exact amount you need to have your baby.......move down and out naturally with ease and with great comfort.......

When you're dilating at 1 cm you become cooler and you allow waves of peace and comfort to flow through you like the gentle movement of the sea.......going back-and-forth allowing......... noticing........ deeper and deeper....... getting nearer and nearer to your call of giving birth...... to a child.........at about 10 cm you know you're in transition where you going to even deep state of relaxation.......... each contraction is like waves of peace and comfort moving through you........ so you may help yourself and your baby to arrive safely and easily.......... at this point you feel the gentle movement of cool air to your body and you allow yourself to settle comfortably........ feeling more comfortable in each moment........ filled with joy and happiness....... going stronger and stronger as you go deeper and deeper.......... helping yourself and your baby knowing the more dilated you are, the more calm and relaxed you are......

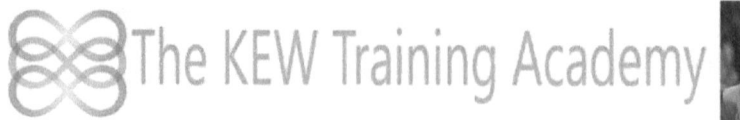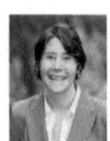

When you become fully dilated you gain more energy...... enthusiasm...... to push your baby into the world at the right time ....you can see your labour coming to completion......... you are aware to push a baby into the world you allow yourself to go into a relaxed state deeper than you've ever been before........ by allowing yourself to go into this state......... you can make your body flow in its natural rhythm helping and assisting the natural movement of your muscles to push your baby into the world......... you relax committing yourself to go deeper and deeper....... the circular muscles of the lower part of the uterus relax allowing the long muscles of the upper part of the uterus to contract and push the baby down the birth canal......... each contraction dilating you gently...... easily ......very quickly....... your birthing muscles will be relaxed at all times....... from the top of your uterus to all the way down to your cervix......

Muscles and tissues remaining completely relaxed....... and dilation taking place very quickly and easily......... so that your cervix is very soft and gently stretches....... perfectly dilating........ to let the baby move down and out easily....... and quickly......... very soft and very stretchy........ you just go deeper and calmer as the head of your baby descends down the birth canal....... you notice more of a desire to push........ you know now that you've been taught how to breathe and you're completely relaxed........

You find having a baby is an accelerated experience because you're so relaxed........ no need to be concerned about moaning which can help to push the baby down........ the pleasure...... the joyful feeling at the moment your baby rotates its head through the cervix and down the vagina........ a wonderfully private and enormously satisfying experience.......... you remain very deeply relaxed...... in control...... feeling calm...... relaxed and strong...... as circular muscles relax...... the long muscles push your baby out and it's a signal for you to go deeper and deeper.......... and this happens so easily.........

You can open our eyes to observe the baby and assist in any way........ feeling calm....... relaxed and confident........ as those muscles relax....... your baby coming into the world....... this is a signal for you to go even deeper with each contraction becoming more calm........ in a more relaxed state of mind becoming stronger....... your body becoming stronger as you go deeper and deeper...... and deeper still........ your uterus works so well bringing your baby down........ and out ....of your pelvis

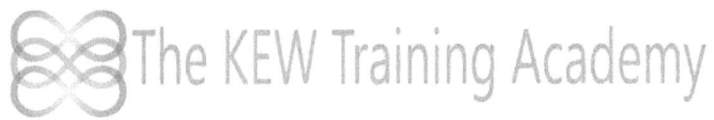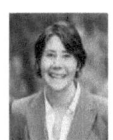

Plenty of room for your baby to be able to pass through……. and you remain in that level of numbness where you feel pressure…. movement no discomfort and you're able to respond to everything in an appropriate manner ……..allowing the time that you need…….. knowing when you need to push your baby to move down and out with ease …….your baby descends to the birthing path ……….visualise your birthing canal opening up……. feeling the gentle movement down through the birth canal……… feeling the movement of your baby's head all around your perineum……. you will remain calm and act appropriately to help yourself and your baby during the birth ……..you're able to assist your baby coming out into the world…….. watching the birth of your baby……. knowing when to open your eyes does not bring you back to your usual state of awareness……… that enables you to feel more calm and relaxed.

When your baby is born your baby's face near you………. you focus all your attention on your baby's face…… eyes……. the babies features……. beautiful features……. bonding ……nurturing…….. your child easily effortlessly……. and naturally able to nurture baby in complete comfort and confidence……….
to continue to relax now as this recording comes to an end and you continue to relax as you put this on repeat and it continues to take you to an even deeper level of relaxation……

BRING OUT OF HYPNOSIS

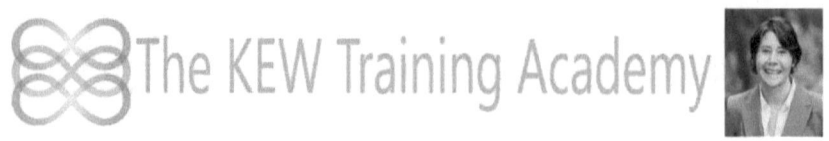

MODULE 6:
THE FINAL ASSESSMENT & OUTLINES FOR YOUR CASE STUDY

One Case Study (written out as the below guidelines and enclosing a recorded session) should be completed and sent to The KEW Training Academy. The recording must include the consultation and the session itself.

YOU MAY CHOOSE TO RECORD ANY SESSION WITH YOUR CLIENT FROM THE SESSIONS YOU DO WITH THEM. YOUR RECORDING MUST BE IN ENGLISH.

Clients name:

Date Of Session:

Prior Hypnosis Experience of Client (If any):

Rapport Level Between Yourself & Client:

Weeks of Client's Gestation:

The Reason The Client Wants Hypnosis for Childbirth:

Session That You Used:

What Stands Out To You About This Client?

What did you learn as the therapist from this session?

What, if anything would you have done differently?

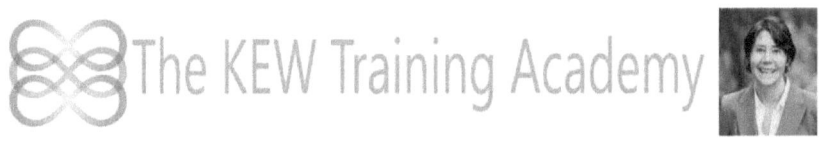
The KEW Training Academy

Thank You

Thank you for participating in this course. If you wish to obtain the Hypnosis for Childbirth Diploma you are required to submit 1 Case Study This case study must include a recorded session of the Hypnosis for Childbirth programme along with written notes as per the outlines in this course. These can be emailed to: hello@kewtraining.com

Thank you and good luck,

Karen E Wells

Co-Founder & Director of The KEW Training Academy Ltd